PREVENTING CAREGIVER BURNOUT

Placement of this book was made
possible by a grant to
LifeTime Resources
from the
Dearborn County Community Foundation

Other books by James R. Sherman, Ph.D.

How to Overcome a Bad Back
How to Survive Rejection and Promote Acceptance
Get Set...GO!
Escape to the Gunflint
Stop Procrastinating: Get to Work
Plan Your Work: Work Your Plan
* Sharpening Your Edge

In the DO IT! Success Series

Stop Procrastinating–DO IT!
Patience Pays Off
No More Mistakes
Plan for Success
Farewell to Fear
Be a Winner

In the Caregiver Survivor Series

Preventing Caregiver Burnout
Creative Caregiving
Positive Caregiver Attitudes
The Magic of Humor in Caregiving
* The Caregiver's Guide to Problem Solving
* Conquering Caregiver Fears
* Strengthening the Caregiver Family
* Love, Companionship, and Caregiving
* Health Strategies for Active Caregivers
* The Caregiver's Need for People
* The Caregiver's Planning Guide
* Financial Fitness for Caregivers

* = books in production

PREVENTING CAREGIVER BURNOUT

James R. Sherman, Ph.D.

Pathway Books

Copyright © 1994 by James R. Sherman, Ph.D.

Library of Congress Catalog Card Number
James R. Sherman
Preventing Caregiver Burnout

International Standard Book Number
0–935538–16–X

Manufactured in the United States of America by Malloy Lithographing, Inc.

Design by Group Design

0 9 8 7 6 5 4 3 2 1

Pathway Books
700 Parkview Terrace
Golden Valley, Minnesota 55416–3439
(612) 377–1521

Dedicated to Caregivers

*"The capacity to care is the thing that
gives life its deepest significance and meaning."*

PREFACE

These books contain a wealth of ideas for caregivers like you who want to learn but have a limited time for reading. Use them as valuable resource guides. Familiarize yourself with the contents as you go through them for the first time, then come back again and again whenever a need arises. Like any good resource, these books will always provide an easy–to–follow solution or tell you where to go to find one.

Have a pen or pencil handy as you read each book and mark the pages that are important to you. Answer the questions that are asked, fill in the lists, and add notes of your own whenever you can expand on a usable idea. Let the books work for you.

Keep in mind that these are self–help books that are going to make you a better caregiver. They'll re–ignite your zest for caregiving and get you feeling good again as long as you keep harvesting the material they contain.

ACKNOWLEDGEMENTS

My wife Merlene has guided me through the complex world of caregiving. She has spent countless hours pulling, pushing, reviewing, editing, and otherwise shaping my thoughts as I wrote these books. It has been said that the supreme test of marriage is when husbands and wives put up wallpaper together. That doesn't stand a candle to writing, editing, designing, printing, and marketing a series of books. I could never in a million years have brought these books to life if it had not been for her help.

Special thanks go to Chris Sherman, our eldest son, editor, and friend. Like his brothers, Eric and Lincoln, he is doing everything he can to bring us into the 21st century.

I would also like to thank Bruce Eaton, Lisa Haines and Lori Anderson at Group Design, Jim Thalhuber and Kay Cady at Courage Center, Etta Erickson and Dr. Edward Ratner of the Abbott–Northwestern Hospital Geriatric Team, the folks at Senior Resources, Edna Ballard, Joan Bowlin, Carol Bratter, Bev Colson, Rev. Dr. Ed Daniel, Audrey De La Martre, Thelma Edwards, Carol Feldheim, Lynn Friss Feinberg, Mary Flynn, Karen Hanauer, Sally Hebson, Barbara Heinemann, Dr. Kenneth Hepburn, Betty Kane, Barbara Lepis, Dr. Robert Meiches, Robert Provost, Rev. David Ruhmkorff, Jane Royse, Virginia Schiaffino, Gail Skoglund, Andrea Skolkin, Sandra Varpness, Jean Velleu, Eva Walker, and Nancy Webster for their kind words, support, suggestions, and encouragement.

If there are errors in fact, style, format, or whatever, they are mine to bear.

ENDORSEMENTS

Edna L. Ballard, ACSW, Senior Fellow, Duke University Center for the Study of Aging and Human Development
> " ...written in a straightforward, appealing style that allows caregivers to use the books at their own pace. Dr. Sherman clearly recognizes the many emotional facets of caregiving and offers timely, useful information about coping strategies and caregiving techniques."

Joan Mason Bowlin, Geriatric Nurse Practitioner
> "...a format that provides empowering, interactive reader participation. The Series emphasizes the need for caregivers to take care of themselves."

Carol Bratter, Executive Director, People Helper's Foundation
> "Caregivers who are energy–depleted and time–deprived will find this series useful, concise, practical, and relevant. A must for caregiver– volunteer training."

Bev Colson and Carol Feldheim, cofounders, Altercare, Inc. Adult Daycare
> "Packed full of strategies for special people who care."

The Reverend Dr. C. Edwin Daniel, United Methodist Minister
> "Every caregiving person and organization that has responsibility for a care receiver will be helped greatly in their ministry by reading and rereading each book in the Caregiver Survival Series. The books are caring, creative, positive, uplifting, and intelligently honest."

Lynn Friss Feinberg, Family Caregiver Alliance

"The Caregiver Survival Series should prove useful and invaluable to caregivers. It adds to the caregiving literature by providing practical advice and clearly defined steps for caregivers to follow."

Mary Flynn, social worker and caregiver of a stroke survivor

"...a dynamite tool for teaching...lots of material...excellent resource for workshops or study guide for support groups. This series is loaded with ideas to help caregivers take control and take care of their lives."

Karen Hanauer, Employee Assistance Counselor, Cargill, Inc.

" ...inspiring guidelines for employee assistance counselors...packed with tangible tools and indispensible resources for corporations that are involved with employee eldercare issues."

Robert K. Meiches, M.D. Geriatrician

"The Caregiver Survival Series is an excellent resource for caregivers...full of practical and accurate information. It's a needed and valuable new caregiver resource."

Reverend David Ruhmkorff, Episcopal priest

"A series that's almost custom designed for the ministry. A caregiving encyclopedia to help caregivers help themselves."

Gail Skoglund, Social Worker, Intergenerational Daycare

"Our support groups hunger for the concrete caregiving ideas and strategies that overflow from this series."

Andrea Skolkin, Director, Metropolitan Area Agency on Aging, Minneapolis and St. Paul

"The dynamic self–help concepts and solutions encompass a multitude of intergenerational caregiving issues for caregivers in all walks of life."

Sandra Varpness, Social Worker, Methodist Hospital's Parkinson's Center

"The thought–provoking questions in each section lend a fresh approach for counseling and caregiver support group discussions."

Elva D. Walker, Previous Chair, National Council on Aging

"Dr. Sherman clearly articulates the complexities of caregiving and follows up with clues, answers, and strategies to help give readers a meaningful and satisfying caregiving role."

Nancy B. Webster, caregiver for her octogenarian mother

"...an uplifting treasury of practical information for those of us who care deeply about our loved ones and want to maintain a sense of perspective while giving care."

TABLE OF CONTENTS

PICTURE YOURSELF IN THIS SITUATION

☞ You feel physically, emotionally, and psychologically exhausted. You're under constant stress in an intense caregiving relationship that fails to produce the kind of change or recovery you're hoping for.

☞ You've lost your intensity and incentive and are weighed down by increasing emotional pressure. You're facing four common dilemmas that are often felt by overworked caregivers.

✔ You find little satisfaction in caregiving.
✔ You must force yourself to do routine caregiving tasks.
✔ You feel listless and in need of diversion.
✔ You feel a growing need to be someplace else.

1

Do you fit this model? If you do, you're a candidate for *caregiver burnout.*

"WHOA! Me? What are you talking about?"

You just read a general description of caregiver burnout. It's neither a physical ailment nor a neurosis, even though it has both physical and psychological aspects. One of the great costs of burnout is the loss of truly effective service by some of society's very best people. That includes you.

You don't have to go through burnout, nor does anyone else. The purpose of this book is to demonstrate why caregivers get burned out and what can be done to prevent it. You'll learn about the process of caregiving and the people who are doing it. You'll also see what causes caregiver burnout.

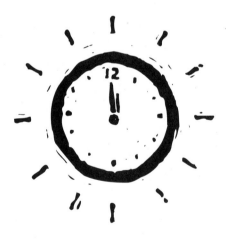

THE NATURE OF CAREGIVING

Pablo Casals, the world renowned cellist, said, *"The capacity to care is the thing that gives life its deepest significance and meaning."*

WHO ARE YOU?

As a caregiver, you're one of thousands of courageous people who provide for the daily needs of disabled or chronically ill family members or friends. You do so in a way that enables them to live at home. In addition to providing physical comfort and safety, you also help preserve your care receiver's dignity and self–esteem.

Caregiving is not just hand–holding. It's difficult and exhausting work. Like most caregivers, you probably help with cooking, cleaning, laundry, and shopping. You provide transportation and run errands. You're responsible for personal care and hygiene, including bathing, dressing, grooming, and toileting. You often coordinate medical care and assistance, give medications, and change dressings or intravenous tubes.

No type of care is exempt from your hands. No chore is too basic. In a single day your responsibilities may range from doing the wash and cleaning the house to buying groceries and filling out reimbursement forms. You learn to eat and sleep when your care receiver eats and sleeps, and you hurry to accomplish everything else in the time between.

You provide emotional support and companionship and are usually the one who makes decisions about personal and household finances. You almost always get involved in care that is provided by speech, physical, or occupational therapists and public health nurses.

On top of all that, you're called upon to supply up–to–date information to friends, loved ones, other family members, and health professionals.

HOW DO YOU COMPARE?

At times, you may feel isolated from other people because you think your caregiving circumstances set you apart from others. But in reality, you're probably not much different than thousands of other caregivers. Here are some characteristics of the group to which you belong.

Common Characteristics of Caregivers

- You're probably a "primary caregiver," which means you're basically in charge of everything that happens to your care receiver.

- As a primary caregiver, you get little or no help from anyone else. The help you do get comes from family or friends.

- If you're a family caregiver, you provide about 80% of all personal and medically–related care and about 90% of all home–help services.

- Most likely, you're caring for your spouse. If you're not a spouse, you're probably a son, daughter, or daughter–in–law.

- You could be anywhere from 21 to 90 years of age. The average age of all caregivers is in the mid–fifties.

- You've possibly had some previous, short–term experience giving care to a friend, family member, or loved one.

- If you're an average caregiver, you're spending four hours a day, seven days a week with your care receiver. If your care receiver is severely impaired, you could be spending over 40 hours a week giving heavy–duty care and be on–call 24 hours a day.

- If you're a family caregiver, you're more than likely employed. That means you have to use a lot of creativity to balance your work and home responsibilities with your caregiving duties.

- You're also concerned about your own health, and you should be with all the work you have to do!

WHY DO YOU DO IT?

You have many reasons for providing home care. The most frequent reason is love for your friend or family member and a desire to provide care in familiar surroundings. It could be that home care is your only option, because outside care, even if it's available, is too expensive. You might also be motivated by a sense of obligation, or a concern that no one else can provide the same quality care.

You became a caregiver in one of two ways: (a) you chose to do it, or (b) you had no choice. If it was your choice, you probably based your decision on whether you had the time, energy, money, or patience to do it.

If you had no choice, you probably found yourself suddenly and unexpectedly in a position that demands great personal sacrifice. You may be giving care because of a family commitment, limited financial resources, your proximity to the care receiver, or lack of anyone else to do the job. When you started caregiving, you may have been confused by feelings of guilt or obligation, and you may still have a hard time sorting through those feelings.

In any case, you're doing the best you can by relying on your experience, intuition, and the advice of others. Like it or not, you know you have to make the best of a difficult situation and do what works for you and your care receiver.

GOOD NEWS

The good news is that most caregiving relationships are highly successful. To no one's surprise, most of you are very devoted to your care receivers. You think of them as people and not as adversaries or burdens.

You probably find the role rewarding, and would not think of having it any other way. Still, it isn't easy. It can be physically and emotionally stressful, not only for you, but also for your care receiver.

Caregiving can send your emotions on a roller coaster. Within one day's time you can easily experience rage, fear, hope, sadness, humor, grief, bravery, fatigue, dedication, vigorous advocacy, and most of all, love.

The rage some of you feel is often directed toward what you see as unsympathetic medical or governmental agencies that disregard your care receiver's needs in favor of financial, administrative, and bureaucratic red tape. Sometimes the anger is justified.

Caregiver burden is the term used to refer to the physical, emotional, financial, and psychological problems that can victimize caregivers like you. When the burden becomes too great, it leads to caregiver burnout. That's what happened to Stephanie Ward.

THE BURNOUT OF STEPHANIE WARD

Stephanie Ward is a middle–aged, midwestern housewife and mother of three college–aged children. She is the primary caregiver for her fifty–three year–old husband, Jack, who had a stroke three years ago.

Stephanie's caregiving responsibilities were thrust upon her without warning on the day Jack collapsed at work. Like many other caregivers, she got some information from doctors and discharge planners at the hospital, but had no real concept of what the future would be like.

She was determined to give Jack the best care possible and was very optimistic about potential outcomes. But over time, and in spite of Jack's slow improvement, she began to feel she had nothing to show for her backbreaking efforts. Her feelings of dedication, accomplishment, and self–fulfillment have slowly been replaced by physical, emotional, and mental exhaustion. Her attitude has changed from positive and caring to negative and uncaring.

Stephanie's case holds many of the elements that affect countless other caregivers. You may not have faced the same dilemmas Stephanie has, but you may have encountered others that were just as frustrating. As you go through this book, and read about people like Stephanie, think of the pressures you're facing, jot them down as they come to mind, and look for better ways of defusing them.

STAGES OF BURNOUT

Like many others, Stephanie has gone through what most experts recognize as the three major stages of burnout. See if her experiences are similar to yours.

Stage One – Frustration

Stephanie's repeated disappointments over a perceived lack of progress and her lack of knowledge of what to expect have led to her frustration. Her initial dedication was fueled by the thought that if she tried hard enough, Jack would be like he was before the stroke. When she saw that her efforts produced little change, she ran out of energy and became disenchanted. She came down with more colds and headaches than usual. Insomnia and backaches appeared more frequently and a general feeling of uneasiness set in.

Stephanie began to do what many exhausted caregivers do. She overate and let her physical condition deteriorate. She deceived herself by unwittingly selecting alcohol as a means of escape. This only intensified her frustration. She wasn't burned out yet, just a little singed around the edges.

> *Research has shown that caregivers like Stephanie report three times as many stress symptoms as the general population. They take more over–the–counter and prescription drugs to help cope with the psychological strains of caregiving. They also lose interest in social and recreational activities and are less likely to seek companionship or join support groups.*

Stage Two – Depression

In Stage Two, Stephanie was besieged by prolonged grief and periodic depression. She cried a lot and didn't know why.

She thought her efforts were being second–guessed by family and friends and felt hurt by their suggestions or constructive criticisms. She got angry and bitter, especially toward Jack, who she felt was the cause of all her problems. She sometimes overreacted with outbursts of hostility and told Jack, *"I wouldn't be in this mess if it weren't for you"*.

Stephanie grew inflexible. She felt that **her** way was the only way out of her predicament, and she resented any suggestions to the contrary.

Stephanie could have recovered at this point, gained control of her caregiving problems, avoided Stage Three (total burnout), and found satisfaction from the events that made it challenging. To do so, she would have had to recognize and deal with her fatigue and restore the positive attitudes she had when she started giving care.

She needed to reach out to friends, relatives, neighbors, or caregiver support groups who understood her dilemmas. She could have done it by herself, but it would have been a lot easier if she had someone helping her.

Stage Three – Despair

Stephanie is now in the final stage of burnout, feeling helpless and adrift. She has lost her concentration and effectiveness, makes more mistakes, and is unable to get excited about any progress Jack might make. Caregiving has become mechanical and enforced. Devotion has been replaced by cynicism. Negative reactions have been replaced by feelings of hopelessness. Her heart is no longer in giving care.

Like many other burned–out caregivers, Stephanie frequently skips routine tasks like bathing, fixing her hair, or changing clothes. Personal accomplishments are few and far between.

Stephanie has lost her sense of humor. She can't laugh at herself, at the tragic reality of her situation, or at things that other people think are funny. She is indifferent to the happiness of others, and finds no joy in books, television, or movies. She sees nothing but drudgery in her life.

Stephanie has lost interest in her church, community, and social groups. She keeps to herself and rarely sees close friends and family. She's tired of being known as the "caring spouse," and is no longer interested in what other people think about her. She has gradually become inaccessible to those who are trying to help.

> It's ironic that burnout, which supposedly comes from intense interaction with other people, can get worse when a person is alone and has nobody around to provide support.

THE BOTTOM LINE

The most notable thing about Stephanie's experience is that it has gone on for as long as it has without her realizing what was happening. She hasn't recognized the symptoms and is too upset to hear about them from someone else.

Stephanie's feelings of anger, frustration, anxiety, and depression are common responses to uncommon stress. In most cases, the negative feelings are temporary, specific, and localized. But with burned–out caregivers, the feelings are generalized and occur more frequently until they become chronic.

Burnout raises lots of red flags for you and others to see. Recognize them early, deal with them decisively, and burnout may be prevented. Here are some things to watch out for:

✔ alienation
✔ irritability

✔   impatience
✔   withdrawal
✔   lack of compassion
✔   sensitivity to criticism
✔   loss of hope, purpose, and meaning

It's not uncommon for the stages of burnout to overlap. The important thing to remember is that any combination of feelings and experiences can result in burnout if the caregiver or someone else fails to recognize them in time to intervene.

CAUSES AND CURES

Stephanie Ward's is a classic case of caregiver burnout, but she is not alone. Many people have fallen into the same predicament. This book describes in detail some of the devastation caregiver burnout can cause. It gets a little heavy at times, but that's the nature of burnout. Read it carefully, and learn what causes burnout by witnessing how other caregivers have struggled through its early stages. Discover the variety of strategies you can use to make sure burnout doesn't undermine your caregiving efforts.

In the section that follows, you'll find brief accounts of some of the major causes of burnout. Read them all, answer the questions they pose, and try to relate each case to your own situation.

Once you know what causes burnout, you'll be better prepared to avoid it. The last two sections of this book will build on your understanding of the problem and provide the strategies you need to be a happy and successful caregiver.

"Better by far you should forget and smile, than that you should remember and be sad." – Christina Georgina Rossetti, English poet.

THE CAUSES OF CAREGIVER BURNOUT

Why did Stephanie Ward suffer burnout?

✔ She got frustrated and confused as her role as caregiver changed over time.
✔ She was affected by hidden factors that seemed to be out of her control.
✔ She failed to realize that her dilemmas were not unlike those faced by other caregivers who suffered burnout.

CHANGING ROLES

Some of you are confused about your roles. You're filled with feelings of love and compassion for your care receiver, and you feel you should share your care receiver's suffering. You also know you should take an objective approach to the treatment of the disability.

You're frustrated because you don't think you're providing adequate care. Those of you who practice "tough love" can separate your role as spouse, lover, and friend from your role as rehabilitative caregiver. Others cannot. It's a difficult dilemma that many caregivers just can't handle.

HIDDEN FACTORS

Some of you are either unable or unwilling to recognize shortcomings which are *not your fault*. Your predisposition to burnout may be a factor of your age, sex, physical stature, psychological makeup, or other inherited characteristics that you're not aware of. You continue to give care without a break until you are physically and mentally spent. If you can't get help, you eventually reach the point where you can no longer continue.

Most underlying causes of burnout come directly from the nature of caregiving. It's a balancing act between tasks and responsibilities on one hand, and self–esteem, coping skills, and social support on the other. The demands are excruciating.

BRIEF ACCOUNTS

Here are ten accounts that describe how some people got caught up in the early stages of caregiver burnout. Read each account carefully, and then try to answer the questions that follow. Your answers will give you insight into your own feelings about caregiving and the causes of burnout.

You will also discover, as you go through the accounts, that creative ideas will pop into your head for improving your own caregiving situation. Write your ideas down as they come to mind and add them to the suggestions and strategies that are provided. The more you know about burnout and the ways to prevent it, the stronger you'll be if you run into problems later.

Some of the best remedies can be gathered from doctors, nurses, therapists, psychologists, members of the clergy, family members, or close friends. Keep in mind the suggestions those folks provide as you work your way through these accounts. Don't hesitate to add those suggestions to your arsenal of ideas.

When you finish reading each account, write down in the space provided how you would solve the problems that are presented. It will get you primed for working out your own strategies later on.

☐ UNREALISTIC EXPECTATIONS

Aaron Segal is a prime candidate for burnout because of the expectations he has for himself, his wife Polly who is dying from AIDS, and the caregiving situation that binds them together. He gets very frustrated when his expectations of what he and others should think and do fail to materialize. The more he expects, the more frustrated he becomes when his expectations are not met.

Here are some of the expectations Aaron shares with many other disappointed caregivers.

- ✔ Expecting immediate success.
- ✔ Expecting Polly to be more motivated.
- ✔ Expecting others to be more understanding.
- ✔ Expecting to know how to handle every situation.
- ✔ Expecting regular appreciation and positive comments from Polly.
- ✔ Expecting that the caregiving experience will work a miracle in his own life.
- ✔ Expecting that his caregiving efforts will decisively alter the course of Polly's condition.
- ✔ Expecting specific caregiving tasks and useful feedback on how he's doing from doctors and family.

> *Aaron should try to differentiate between what he hopes will happen, based on his desires, and what is likely to happen, based on increased knowledge and experience. Aaron can bridge the gap by joining an AIDS family support group where he can communicate with and learn from other caregivers who share similar concerns.*

How do you handle emotional distress when your caregiving expectations are not met?

My Thoughts: _____

_____

☐   UNREALISTIC GOALS

Ramon Padilla, who is a single parent, provides care for his teenage son who suffered a fractured skull and brain damage in a boating accident. He gets most of his information about caregiving through trial and error. Since the accident, in which his wife was killed, Ramon has muddled through, as best he could, not knowing what to expect. He is continually surprised and disappointed when setbacks occur. He doesn't know how to prevent them or what to do when he encounters them.

Ramon has no idea of the severity of his son's head injury, nor is he realistic about what he can expect to gain from his caregiving efforts. He thinks only in terms of total recovery and fails to recognize improvements that his son or professional caregivers feel excited about.

Ramon is discovering how hard it is to be both a parent and a caregiver, and it bothers him. But instead of trying to learn more about caregiving, he spends much of his time in fruitless pursuits, most of which are unrelated to his son's condition or to the fundamentals of caregiving. It seems that his major concern is trying to assess blame for the accident, rather than caring for one of its victims.

> *To avoid burnout, Ramon should try to better understand his son's disability and his own ability to deal with it. With the help of health care professionals and other caregivers, he can direct his efforts toward identifiable and achievable goals and objectives. Once he gets some solid direction, his frustration will fade and burnout will become less of a threat.*

What yardstick do you use in evaluating your caregiving effectiveness? Do you work from a set of goals or objectives?

My Thoughts: _____

_____

☐ LACK OF CONTROL

Helen Loos knows that her husband Duane's depression is widespread and long–lasting. She also knows she can't turn back the clock and make things the way they used to be before Duane became ill. That leaves her sad and frustrated, because the situation seems to be totally out of her control.

Helen's perceived helplessness is further compounded by what she sees as major obstacles, including a lack of finances, few willing volunteers, little professional assistance, no support from family members, lack of planning and scheduling skills, and poor organizational and time–management skills. She tries to be upbeat so she doesn't upset Duane. She's afraid that her hopelessness will only make him feel worse.

What Helen thought would be short–term caregiving has unexpectedly become long–term. She now knows that she's in over her head, but she doesn't know how she can cut back on her efforts. Especially since she feels she is solely responsible for every caregiving task.

The deeper Helen gets into caregiving, the more she tries to escape. The continuous demands have worn her down and left her physically and emotionally exhausted. She feels her situation is so hopeless that no one else would be willing to help her.

Helen's susceptibility toward burnout can be halted once she recognizes that other people are available to help in each of her problem areas. Only after she makes a move to seek out and start drawing on the expertise of others will she regain control of her life.

What steps have you taken to gain some measure of control over your caregiving responsibilities?

My Thoughts: _____

_____

☐ OVERLOAD

When Peter Richards' wife Angela was diagnosed with multiple sclerosis, Peter willingly assumed her care, but now he has second thoughts. He feels that no matter how hard he works, there is no end in sight, nothing has been gained, and he sees no respite from his caregiving chores. He's wearing himself out and doesn't think either he or Angela is making progress. He can only accept the hard work of caregiving as long as he feels he is gaining ground, controlling the outcome, and being rewarded for his efforts. But the outcomes and rewards are not always there, and without that feeling of satisfaction, he's courting burnout.

Angela, who has always been frail, has appreciated the help that Peter has always given her. Now, being depressed, and *needing* Peter's help, she has become very demanding. The strain between them is growing every day.

Peter sees no end to the care he gives, it just seems to go on forever, without change. He faces the same tasks day in and day out, like being in the army and peeling an endless supply of potatoes.

Unfortunately, Peter has placed unreasonable demands on himself. He discourages others from giving help and insists on carrying the entire load single–handedly. He is very rigid in his approach and finds it difficult to adjust to new situations. He has sought no substitutes or diversions from his caregiving tasks, so now he is locked into a never–ending role that has few opportunities for respite. He's in a rut and no longer motivated to seek new challenges or new directions. The more he overextends himself, the more uptight he becomes, and the more likely he is to snap.

> *Peter needs respite from his caregiving. Either he has to recognize that he needs help before he burns out, or someone close to him must tell him what is happening. He can, if he asks for it, find respite through friends, neighbors, volunteers, or adult daycare centers.*

How do you think caregiving can be changed for people like Peter who see it as being tedious, uninteresting, without variety, and offering no rewards or incentives?

My Thoughts: _____

_____

☐   CRITICISM FROM OTHERS

Martha Weber has no defense against her well–intentioned relatives, friends, and onlookers who are always ready with unsolicited advice or criticism about her caregiving. Their pointed remarks have gently but sadly intensified her anxieties and conflicts. She is especially susceptible to spontaneous comments about how bad her husband Frank looks and seems to feel.

Martha already knows a lot about Frank's throat cancer, and she knows she is doing the best she can. But the negative reminders suggest that she is still not doing enough. She feels that the people who are criticizing her are actually saying they could do it better than she can. It's ironic, because she's a 24–hour–a–day caregiver, while her critics rarely spend more than an hour a week with Frank.

Criticism hits Martha particularly hard, because she is already plagued by several obstacles. Frank's first wife of 36 years died the year before he married Martha. She has never been totally accepted by Frank's family, which puts added stress on her. She has set unrealistic caregiving goals and tends to punish herself when those goals are not met. She is apprehensive in new situations and sometimes lets her emotions get the best of her. She is also excessively concerned with the opinions of other family members. That's a heavy load for anyone.

> *Martha would feel better about herself if she spent time with a counselor, a comforting friend or a support group that can give her positive reinforcement. Regular reminders that she is doing the best she can would help restore her self–esteem and improve her ability to weather criticism from others.*

How have you handled criticism? Do you ignore it or allow it to change your caregiving strategy?

My Thoughts: _____

_____

☐   **ISOLATION**

Estelle Barnard was thrust into caregiving when her 70–year–old father Willis broke his hip in a farm accident. As the only daughter, and the one who took care of her dad after her mother died, she was designated by her siblings as the best suited to provide care. She had previously enjoyed social contacts, but now she has become isolated on the family farm because of her unwavering commitment to her caregiving duties.

Her days seem to drag on as she struggles with boredom, mental stagnation,and the increasing demands of her father. She is tired of having no one but her father to talk to, and there is evidence to suggest that he is tired of it too.

Estelle's social isolation leaves her without a break or outside stimulation. She needs feedback to know if she is doing the right things. Her lack of self–confidence often leads to mistakes and misunderstandings, which in turn lead to frustration and depression.

> *Estelle needs to take a more lighthearted approach toward herself, her father, and the people from whom she has become separated. She can't wait for others to come to her. She has to develop a plan that will ensure outside contacts and still allow private moments in which to grow and pursue her own interests.*

How has your caregiving been affected by the abundance–or the lack–of social contact?

My Thoughts: _____

_____

☐ FINANCIAL DEMANDS

Gretchen Harvey is having a difficult time coping with the financial cost of caregiving. She gave up her job to care for her husband Roy, who can't work because of advanced stages of Parkinson's disease. Since neither of them is working, they've lost income, benefits, and pensions and have had to get by on savings and disability payments.

They are on reduced, fixed incomes, and because of that, have lost much of their real purchasing power. They also had to modify their home to accommodate Roy's disabilities, and are afraid he may someday need to move to a nursing home.

Gretchen doesn't know how long they will be able to meet the mounting costs for doctors, nurses, medications, medical insurance, special equipment, and occupational and physical therapists. She also has to deal with the cost of respite care and home health aides. Roy is worried too, and saddened that he can no longer provide a steady income. He sometimes feels that Gretchen is blaming him for their financial difficulties.

Gretchen's fear of running out of money may or may not be realistic. So far, she has been able to get additional help from tax breaks, family income, and from property she and Roy own together. Her worries about money, when added to her "normal" caregiver burden, can very easily make her another casualty of burnout.

Where would you turn for help if you suddenly found that your funds were running out?

> *Gretchen should talk to a financial advisor that she can trust. If a financial advisor determines that funds are not adequate, she could pursue sources with the help of a social worker. She can locate additional help through family, friends, a local support group, or a social service agency.*

My Thoughts: _____

_____

☐   **PANIC**

Mary Parker became a caregiver after her husband George was involved in a major automobile accident. George suffered a serious head injury and a fractured pelvis, which have kept him incapacitated and bedridden. Mary's initial response was one of panic, because George had always been the dominant force in their marriage. He had always handled their finances. He paid all the bills, took care of their health and accident insurance, and made sure that Mary always had enough money to meet her needs. Mary's panic was heightened by the fact that she hadn't driven a car for years and now felt very isolated.

Panic is a common response that generally subsides as soon as help is available. Mary's panic has continued unabated for many reasons. She doesn't recognize the help that's available, and she lacks the confidence she needs to take charge. She's afraid of being rejected by George because she can't provide the care he needs nor can she get a handle on their financial situation. She's particularly afraid that George might not survive because of something she may or may not do. She's afraid that no one will be around to help her through her most difficult moments. And she is afraid of what other people think of her caregiving.

Whenever Mary runs into an obstacle, no matter how insignificant, she overspends her emotional reserve and panic again sets in. At times, she has even suffered serious panic attacks.

> *Mary can begin to conquer her overpowering fright by building her self–confidence through recognition of the positive things she's accomplishing. She can seek confirmation of her caregiving efforts by establishing a self–reward system and reaching out to other people for additional assurance. Once she does that, she'll gain control of her emotions and be better able to assume command of her caregiving responsibilities.*

How would you handle the panic and fear that is frequently a major factor in caregiving?

My Thoughts: _____

_____

☐   GRIEF

Judy Willis' grief over her husband's Alzheimer's disease is another common response to illness or disability. It often follows panic and usually lasts longer.

Both Judy and Ben feel a sense of loss, because Ben is now physically and mentally impaired. Their loss causes grief. They grieve for the loss of the person Ben used to be before his illness, and they grieve for the loss of a life they were living together before the illness occurred. The world has become quite different for both of them. They can no longer go together on the camping trips they once enjoyed, nor can they go on the worldwide tours they often took with Ben's professional group.

Judy has had a hard time controlling her grief. She doesn't know how or when to express it or whether she should keep it hidden. She doesn't want to upset Ben or make it hard for the friends who come to help. Her emotional turmoil is devastating. Her despair is caused by many of the same feelings that bring on panic attacks.

Judy can help to ease her pain by learning more about her new role as caregiver and understanding the stages of grief she is now experiencing. Social workers, caregiver support groups, health care professionals and others who have had similar experiences can all provide answers to many of Judy's concerns. A daily exercise program would help her feel more mentally and physically fit.

How would you resolve Judy's grief over the loss of "what once was" so she can come to terms with the demands of caregiving?

My Thoughts: _____

_____

☐ DENIAL

Esther Cline's husband Nathan is getting worse instead of better. No matter how hard she works or how skilled she is in giving care, Nathan keeps losing ground from coronary artery disease.

Esther is not doing so well either. She tires quickly. Many times she can't take care of Nathan's needs. This is frustrating for any caregiver, but it is especially stressful for Esther. She stoutly denies the physical and mental changes in Nathan that are now too obvious to be overlooked. She even denies the changes that are the result of aging. She thinks Nathan is in better shape than he says he is, and believes he can do more to help himself. She's having a hard time dealing with a caregiving situation that is wearing her out. Her fatigue and the stress brought on by her denial of Nathan's condition continue to build.

Esther's anger and frustration are also building. To her, Nathan's loss of strength and endurance is not part of a natural process but a direct consequence of her caregiving. She tries to compensate by doing more, and that puts a drain on her own physical and mental stamina. She is experiencing the early stages of caregiver burnout.

> *Esther needs to get a better grasp of her caregiving responsibilities and her ability to handle them. Once she understands the full implications of Nathan's illness, and accepts his and her fatigue, she'll have a more realistic idea of what lies ahead for both of them.*

What part of your care receiver's condition has been the hardest for you to accept?

My Thoughts: _____

_____

TAKE A BREAK

You probably came up with several ideas of your own on how to prevent burnout as you read through the major causes of caregiver burnout. Take a minute now and expand on those ideas. Think of ways of applying what you've discovered to your own caregiving situation. Then go on to the next section, where you'll find twenty–one specific techniques that will make you a better caregiver and help you avoid caregiver burnout.

Combine the following strategies with your own ideas. Match those you think will work best against the causes that bother you the most. Lighten up, get some rest, exercise, or build a support system. Do whatever suits your needs. You won't find all the answers here, but you'll get enough ideas to help you avoid the problems that lead to burnout. And if you can think of some strategies that aren't listed here, write them down in the space provided and use them whenever you can do so.

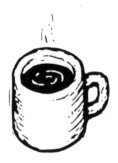

AN OUNCE OF PREVENTION

The first stage of caregiver burnout usually comes on unexpectedly, because caregivers like you don't generally think about being emotionally exhausted. You probably hold to the same high expectations you had when you began caregiving and feel you can handle any problem that crosses your path. Think about your situation as you read through each of the following strategies. Test them against your own feelings and see how close you really are to the edge.

These strategies will prevent burnout or stop it once it has started. You'll find techniques that will show you how to avoid physical and emotional exhaustion. You'll also learn how to recognize and deal with any symptoms that might already be affecting your behavior. If you think you're edging your way into stage–one frustration, admit that something is wrong and figure out which of the following suggestions you can use right now to correct it. Do it now, because if you wait for an easier time, indecision and delay will compound your worries and make things worse.

Get rid of those feelings of guilt or embarrassment about being susceptible to burnout. Divert your energies from anxiety and frustration to practical strategies that will help you cope. It won't be an easy task, but the results will more than outweigh the effort.

Take positive steps now to reduce your frustrations and regain your motivation. As you read through each of the following strategies, make a note to yourself telling how you would apply the suggestions that are given. Start by putting yourself under the microscope.

■ KNOW YOURSELF

"Never lose sight of this important truth, that no one can be truly great until they have gained a knowledge of themselves." Johann Zimmerman, Swiss physicist.

Recognize your talents and skills and put them to good use. If you can play a musical instrument, share your talent with others, especially your care receiver. Music has amazing therapeutic powers, and you can benefit as much as the person you care for.

Accept limitations if you have them, but don't let them hold you back. If you're a lousy cook, admit it and learn to prepare better meals. Seek the help of a nutritionist or someone you know who is a better cook. Don't rely solely on junk food.

Balance your abilities against the nature of caregiving and figure out what is possible and what is not. Talk to other caregivers and see what it takes to be effective. If you can't lift your care receiver, then work out an alternative that will protect your back and still meet your care receiver's needs. Build a hoist, enlist someone to help, or try some other creative solution.

Bask in the glow of past successes and recall failures with a willingness to forgive. If you did a good job raising your family, transfer those skills to caregiving. If you made some mistakes along the way, set them aside and adopt a positive attitude.

Look for patterns of improvement and incorporate them where they will do the most good. If you notice your overall stress level going down, figure out what you're doing right and apply that strategy to all stress–provoking areas.

Keep a written "victory list" of the accomplishments that have given you the most satisfaction. Include graduations, job promotions, and child rearing. Haul out your old golf trophies, county fair awards, or military commendations. List some of the creative things you did to make caregiving easier. Recall the time you brought a smile to your care receiver's face.

MY VICTORY LIST

☺
☺
☺
☺
☺

Review your victory list from time to time to remind yourself that you have succeeded in the past and can succeed again in the future. Consider the courage, patience, and perseverance that helped you then and apply those same skills now.

Analyze your emotions and know how they have influenced you over the years. Emphasize positive feelings, because they are your greatest source of motivation. Search for a better understanding of who you are and what you're trying to do as a caregiver.

My Strategy: _____

_____

■   **TAKE A REALITY CHECK**

Reality checks promote self–awareness by helping to identify the source and effects of stress in caregiving. They're easy to construct and only require a few basic questions. Here's an example, with some sample responses in italics.

Your response to a reality check should provide a good perspective of your caregiving and what you expect from your efforts. The next step is to compare your responses to the way other caregivers feel. Talk to a social worker or a caregiver support group. If you're in a stressful situation, it may be due to your concept of reality. Periodic reality checks like this provide an effective tool for revaluating your caregiving goals.

My Strategy: _____

_____

MY REALITY CHECK

✔ Why am I giving care?
(Because I'm the only one who can do it.)

✔ How does my caregiving reflect who I am, as a unique person?
(I'm the spouse of a stroke survivor.)

✔ Are there ways I can personalize my caregiving, even more than I do now?
(I can use my talents as a singer.)

✔ How concerned am I about personal recognition from family, friends, and others?
(I'll do my best and let the chips fall where they may.)

✔ What recognition do I seek for my efforts?
(Just some warm fuzzies at the end of the day.)

✔ How can I satisfy myself and reduce my reliance on external rewards?
(By reaching my personal goals.)

✔ How does my caregiving fit into the relationships I have with family and friends?
(As the "baby" in our family I don't get much respect.)

✔ How does my caregiving affect the relationships I have with my care receiver?
(I feel like a drill sergeant.)

■ **LIGHTEN UP**

Sebastian Chamfort, the French satirist, said, *"The most utterly lost of all days is one in which you have not once laughed."* He obviously knew the value of laughter in relieving caregiver stress.

A good laugh is more than just a great tension reliever as you can see from the following list. A good laugh...

>   ... aids digestion
>   ... raises your pulse rate
>   ... improves concentration
>   ... strengthens your muscles
>   ... lowers your blood pressure
>   ... activates the creative center of your brain
>   ... stimulates your heart and endocrine system

Three to five minutes of hearty laughter is the equivalent of three strenuous minutes on a rowing machine.

The deeper the giggles, the greater the exercise of internal muscles in your lungs and abdomen. A hearty dose of laughter will do wonders to relieve your assorted aches and pains.

Joy and laughter affect the way you feel about caregiving and, consequently, the way you do it. If you're happy, you'll have fewer problems and will enjoy the pleasure of the person you care for. If you're angry or dissatisfied, your work will drag on, you'll make mistakes, and your care receiver and others will go out of their way to avoid you.

A lighthearted approach to your tasks will increase your creativity, reduce your resistance to change, and provide you with a storehouse of useful ideas. You will feel less threatened by the prospect of stress and find it easier to respond to troublesome demands. All it takes is the ability to see the irony in the painful situations that often characterize caregiving. It might be difficult, but it's up to you. Abraham Lincoln said, *"You're about as happy as you make up your mind to be."*

You can develop a happy, healthy attitude by thinking happy thoughts and doing happy things. Look for happiness in your environment. Read happy books, go to happy movies, watch happy TV. Let your hair down. Allow yourself the pleasure of laughing at things you think are funny.

Take a minute now and make a list of things that have cheered you up and made you happy. Maybe it was a comedy routine by your favorite humorist. Or maybe it was a funny poem you knew as a child. You could include parades, grandchildren, silly jokes, hot fudge sundaes, or old time radio shows; anything that tickles your funny bone.

THINGS THAT I ENJOY

♥ _____

♥ _____

♥ _____

♥ _____

Try to find similar pleasures in your present setting. Look for things you can include as part of your daily life. Share your happy moments with your care receiver and others. You'll find that light–heartedness is not only contagious, it's also good for your health.

My Strategy: _____

_____

■   ACCENTUATE THE POSITIVE

Start each day on a positive note. Pause for a few minutes and write out a statement that expresses the way you would like to feel for the next 24 hours.

> *"I'm raring to go!"*
> *"Hello day! Let's get on with it!"*
> *"This is going to be my lucky day!"*

Describe your most positive state of being. Are you happy? energetic? enthusiastic? full of vim and vitality? Picture yourself as being in that condition throughout the day, particularly when you start feeling downhearted. Don't let your "conservative self" tell you that this is silly. With practice and repetition, it will do wonders.

Give yourself a pep talk and tell yourself why you're a good and capable caregiver. Remind yourself of your strengths and past successes. Recall a challenging task; how overwhelmed you felt and how easy the task now seems in retrospect. (*Like taking your care receiver for a walk for the first time.*) Call a friend and share some "warm fuzzies". (*"My crocuses are blooming!"*)

Be *for* things instead of against things. Play mind games. If a negative thought sneaks into your mind, chase it out with a broom and quickly put a positive thought in its place. Take positive steps to get into a positive frame of mind.

Practice positive self–talk. Get rid of negative words and phrases like, *"I can't," "I won't,"* and *"It's too much to do."* Replace them with, *"I can," "I will,"* and *"It will get done."*

Focus on positive sources of strength. Keep a file of inspirational messages that motivate you and give you good feelings about yourself. Give yourself credit where credit is due.

Feeling good about yourself will make you more acceptant of others. They in turn, will recognize your optimism and will become willing partners in your efforts to be a better caregiver.

List at least four things you did well today and give yourself a star for getting them done.

1. _____ ★

2. _____ ★

3. _____ ★

4. _____ ★

My Strategy: _____

_____

■ **GET RELIEF**

Take a short break from long caregiving sessions whenever you can to refresh your mind and restore your health. The break may last ten minutes or a couple of hours, depending on your caregiving demands, but it needs to be **your** time when you can take care of **your** health needs. Schedule time for rest and relaxation in every day's itinerary, and do something you enjoy.

Relax, meditate, or go for a walk. Read a book, play cards, go golfing, or work in your garden. Talk to a friend, stare out the window, or get some exercise. Chances are, when you get back to the task at hand, you'll be able to take a fresh, new approach to caregiving. If you can share these moments with someone you like, so much the better.

Practice the "relaxation response" that was developed by Dr. Herbert Benson, Associate Professor of Medicine at Harvard University Medical School.

✔   Lie or sit in a comfortable position with your eyes closed.

✔   Let your muscles relax in sequence from your toes up through your face and scalp.

✔   Breathe easily and naturally through your nose.

✔   As you breathe out, silently repeat a word or phrase that will help keep you from being distracted.

Practice this response every day until you can do it effortlessly whenever stress and tension build to unacceptable levels.

Try to take a vacation. It's more than recreation, it's a time of *re–creation* when you can recharge your batteries and get a new outlook on life. If a week is too long, get away for a weekend or a holiday. You're not pampering yourself, you're insuring yourself against burnout. And it's quite possible that your care receiver might like to have some time away from you too.

Relatives, friends, and neighbors are often willing to help when a caregiver needs a vacation. Some home–care services and nursing homes can provide short–term respite care when a caregiver needs a break. Don't hesitate to call on them when you can.

My Strategy: _____

_____

■ GET SMART

The more you know about disabilities, illnesses, and the strategies of caregiving, the more effective you'll be in avoiding caregiver burnout.

Your particular caregiving situation is undoubtedly unique, but other caregivers have probably dealt with some of the same problems and emotions you're facing. Ask them how they deal with stress. Ask them how they can work so hard with so little rest. Find out where they get their caregiving resources. Get as much information as you can, as soon as you can.

If possible, share your caregiving problems with your care receiver. Ask for suggestions on how to make your job easier. Seek to understand your care receiver's feelings and offer to work through mutual problems.

Develop a greater awareness of the illness or disability your care receiver is coping with. Find out from professionals and other caregivers how you and your care receiver will be affected mentally and physically by the need for care. Know what's realistic and what's impossible, considering your care receiver's needs and your ability to handle those needs. Find out where to go for help.

See what services are offered in your community. Look for classes or group meetings that provide educational material or emotional support. If local resources are not available, look for support from national organizations. Each time you reach out to one resource, you will probably find another that is just as helpful in providing assistance.

Check the list of resources starting on page 65. It will give you a good start in your search.

The sooner you understand the ins and outs of caregiving, the better you will be at giving care. Your care receiver will have fewer problems and you'll be less likely to suffer caregiver burnout.

My Strategy: _____

_____

■   **SUBDIVIDE**

If you're overwhelmed by the housework, personal care, and medical assistance that comes with caregiving, subdivide it. Break up each major task into several subtasks that you can complete in fifteen minutes or less. The experience of successfully completing a series of subtasks will leave you with a warm sense of accomplishment. You'll get a lot more done that way, and you'll feel better about doing it. Here's an example:

> *Instead of thinking about a day's worth of housework, break it down into dusting, vacuuming, and picking up. If those categories are still too big, break them down again. Vacuum the living areas, acknowledge your accomplishment, then stop and do something entirely different, like fixing lunch. Then vacuum the bedrooms. Stop again, congratulate yourself, and go to work on another task.*

If you run into a barrier with one subtask, stop. Go to work on another one. Thinking about and completing an entirely different task will give your mind a refreshing break. When you go back to your original problem, you'll probably have a solution that would have been lost if you had sat still and fretted.

Subdividing is particularly effective for unpleasant tasks, because almost anyone can do something they dislike if they only have to do it for a short time. Break down bothersome tasks into smaller subtasks. Spread them out and fill the time between with things you like to do. It may take a little longer, but you'll feel better when you're done.

To keep unpleasant tasks from piling up, assign yourself one "DO IT!" day (or afternoon) each month. Mark the day on your calendar, then spend that time cleaning up troublesome tasks that you've set aside.

My Strategy: _____

_____

■ DO IT BETTER

Add variety to your caregiving by doing things in new and different ways. Get your care receiver involved in changing colors, sounds, and smells by using paints, stereos, and a potpourri. Add variety to common, mundane chores by dressing up or down for special days. Celebrate national holidays with ethnic foods and decorations.

Seek beauty in the things you do. Establish pleasant little rituals like putting a ribbon in your care receiver's hair or putting a flower on your care receiver's breakfast tray. Sing old–time favorites you've both enjoyed. Haul out the photo album.

You might think these rituals sound silly, but they're worth their weight in gold if they keep your spirits up, make your care receiver happy, and eliminate some major causes of burnout.

Balance your caregiving responsibilities against the welfare of the people who depend on you. Look at the sacrifices that are being made by your spouse, your children, your friends, and others. Don't give care at their expense or at the cost of your own physical and mental health. You need time and energy to make yourself and everybody else feel happy.

Eliminate unnecessary tasks, and delegate what you can to family, friends, or helpful neighbors. Call on people who are willing to help with housework, shopping, or tending to your care receiver's personal needs. Seek assistance from your church, volunteer organizations, or public agencies that provide services to caregivers. You may be pleasantly surprised at the number of people who are willing to help.

Use common sense and adapt. If a task cannot be done one way, ask yourself if it could be done differently or not at all. If your care receiver can't handle a fork or spoon, serve finger foods. If sleeping is a problem, stay up and pursue an enjoyable hobby instead of lying in bed and worrying. If you're at the end of your rope, use your imagination to come up with one thing you can change to make life easier. Go to work on it. Once that one is taken care of, move on to something else.

My Strategy: _____

_____

■   PLAN YOUR DAYS

Charles Kettering, onetime chairman of General Motors, was asked why he spent so much time in planning. *"My interest is in the future,"* he said, *"because I'm going to spend the rest of my life there."*

Know what you're going to do, when you're going to do it, and where it will take you when you're finished. Define your goals and objectives early. They are the steppingstones to a favorable future and the footings upon which all caregiving should be based. Without them, you stand little chance of avoiding burnout.

Goals are long–term, idealistic statements of hoped–for accomplishments.

Objectives are clear, concise statements of activities you want to complete in specific time periods.

Milestones are intermediate points you have to reach as you move toward individual objectives.

Your goal may be a desire to get some rest from your caregiving duties. Your objective might be to have lunch with a friend two weeks from today. Milestones for your adventure might be making reservations at your favorite eatery, arranging transportation to and from, and getting someone to stay with your care receiver.

If your milestones are spaced close together, you'll arrive at them sooner and satisfy them quicker. Each successful arrival will boost your morale, give you a greater sense of anticipation, and generate the enthusiasm you'll need to reach your final goal.

Share your goals with friends. They'll keep you on track, assist when they can, and help you celebrate when you reach your hoped–for outcomes.

Here's a handy outline for planning your days, using caregiving as an example. You can also use it to set goals for other important areas of your life, including health, social, family, personal, spiritual, financial, and professional. Make each of your goals specific and measurable. Set a time limit for accomplishing them, and describe the outcomes you intend to achieve. Use a calendar to establish your starting date and don't forget to chart your progress.

PLANNING MY DAYS

Major Caregiving Goal:

Specific Caregiving Objectives:

Milestones:

My Strategy: _____

_____

■ ASSIGN PRIORITIES

Avoid the threat of burnout by staying focused. Know which tasks have to be done right away and which can be done later. Give highest priority to tasks that are important **and** urgent.

A task is **important** if it gets you where you're going and doesn't take an unreasonable amount of time and effort. An **urgent** task is one that calls for immediate action. It could be a complete waste of time. *(Your neighbor wants you to run right over to see your local dogcatcher on TV.)*

The *most* important tasks are those that are important **and** urgent, because if you don't do them right away, you'll probably suffer serious consequences. *(Calling 911 when you or your care receiver has chest pains and nausea.)*

Separate your **have to** tasks from your **choose to** tasks. Having to take a break and choosing to go to a ballgame are not the same.

Avoid busy work when you can, and try not to let others waste your time. Don't be afraid to say *"No!"* to unimportant tasks that can disrupt your caregiving strategy.

Reexamine your priorities from time to time so you know you're on the right track and doing the things that benefit you the most. Feel free to change priorities if it looks like things aren't going the way they should.

Sometimes it makes sense to work on a nonessential task that's not as urgent or important as some others. If it doesn't take much time, and if the benefits are substantial, it could serve as a warm–up exercise for more important tasks that could come later. Here are some examples of nonessential tasks that might make you or your care receiver feel better.

✔   Read to your care receiver at breakfast, before an afternoon nap, or in the evening after dinner.
✔   Take your care receiver for an early morning stroll to see the first robins of spring.
✔   Call a close friend first thing in the morning and share some positive thoughts for five or ten minutes.

My Strategy: _____

_____

■   **MANAGE TIME**

Charles Buxton, the English author, wrote, *"You will never find time for anything. If you want time, you must make it."*

Time is a very precious commodity, and once it's gone, you can never get it back. It tells you when some things ought to be done, and reminds you when it's too late to do others. If you don't have a date book to guide your efforts, your caregiving plans may seem like meaningless wanderings through space.

Manage time like money and make every minute count. Keep track of the time you spend and balance your date book like you balance your checkbook. Be sure to set aside prime time for really important tasks.

Be realistic in your time estimates. Know how much caregiving you can provide in a specified time period. Trying to do more than is humanly possible or taking shortcuts can be dangerous to your care receiver's health. Resist the urge to combine incompatible activities, like preparing your care receiver's medications while talking on the phone, in an attempt to save time.

Recognize seasons and cycles, and schedule caregiving activities according to your calendar. Set precise deadlines but allow enough flexibility to take care of unexpected events that can't be postponed.

Don't waste time on things that cause problems or make you feel bad. Lying in the grass and counting daisies is not wasted time if you need a break. Arguing over the price of tea in China is a total loss.

Finally, don't let other people steal your time. It's far too valuable to you and your care receiver, and you'll never get it back.

My Strategy: _____

_____

■ REWARD YOURSELF

The next time you're tempted to throw in the towel, back off, take a deep breath, put a smile on your face, and give yourself a reward for all the good things you've been doing as a caregiver. Reward yourself for bringing an unexpected smile to the face of your care receiver. Reward yourself for coming up with three new ways of preventing caregiver burnout. Give yourself a special bonus for starting an exercise program. Then chalk up a victory in the win column and give yourself a reward for hanging in there.

Self–rewards help build self–confidence. Self–confidence produces optimism and self– control, and optimism and self–control are excellent indicators of a well–adjusted caregiver.

Reward yourself only when you've earned it, but if you've earned it, be sure to take it. A reward system only works when you stick with it.

Your rewards can be simple and inexpensive, but they should be things that are important to you. Pamper yourself with a glass of wine, a hot–fudge sundae, a warm bubble bath, a cup of tea with a friend, a trip to the zoo, or an exciting mystery novel. Try several things until you can find a reward system that will help maintain your confidence and motivation. Make a list now of some of the rewards you'd like to have and the strategy you'd use to get them.

REWARDS I'D LIKE TO HAVE

♥ _____

♥ _____

♥ _____

♥ _____

■ EXERCISE

Nothing can take the edge off a stressful day like exercise. It will give you added energy and allow you to carry out your caregiving tasks in a refreshed and relaxed atmosphere.

Numerous studies have shown that people who exercise as little as 20 minutes a day, three times a week, are less fatigued, can do more work, and are more even–tempered than those who don't exercise.

Exercise doesn't have to be strenuous to be effective. Walking, for example, is considered by most experts to be one of the easiest and best exercises.

Walking is a preventative as well as a remedy for heart, respiratory, and circulation disorders. It actually works as a second heart by expanding and contracting muscles in your feet, calves, thighs, and buttocks. Normally, your heart can propel blood very well on its own. But when the blood transportation system becomes sluggish because of lack of exercise, the heart has to compensate by doing more work. This raises your heart rate and blood pressure. When you walk, the muscles in your lower regions help pump blood back to the heart so it doesn't have to work so hard. That, in turn, lowers your heart rate and blood pressure.

Walking aids digestion, helps elimination, promotes sleep, and is an antidote to physical and psychological tensions. It also helps control weight. It won't take off many pounds, but it will help keep your weight at a desirable level once you've dieted away the excess.

The best time to walk is whenever you can fit it into your caregiving routine. If you walk at a normal pace of three miles an hour, you should be able to walk a mile in about 20 minutes. The best place to walk is wherever it's pleasant and convenient. It could be on the street around your block or in the mall of your neighborhood shopping center. Next time you take your care receiver in for therapy, take your walking shoes along and hike around the medical center.

Be sure to check with your doctor before starting with your exercises.

My Strategy: _____

_____

■ STAY HEALTHY

Good physical health and mental health are absolutely indispensable for preventing caregiver burnout. If you sacrifice your health for the well–being of your care receiver, you will hasten the day when your rundown condition will keep you from providing any care at all. You owe it to yourself and your care receiver to eat properly, exercise regularly, get plenty of sleep, and take an occasional break from your caregiving responsibilities.

You can live a healthy life and prevent physical and emotional exhaustion by eating from the four basic food groups of dairy products, meats and fish, breads and cereals, and fruits and vegetables. Strive for a balanced diet of fats, proteins, carbohydrates, vitamins, minerals, and water. Try to limit your intake of sugar, fat, and salt. Cut down on sweets, no matter how much you crave a chocolate bar. Eat a variety of foods in moderation, and, whenever possible, eat in a relaxed atmosphere.

Be conscious of how much you eat. You increase the risk or severity of a variety of medical problems if you're more than 20 % over your ideal weight. Choose your food wisely, even if you have to give up some longtime favorites like butter, bacon, and beer.

Overwhelming evidence indicates that smoking is one of the leading causes of premature disease and death in this country. It can have a devastating effect on your day–to–day health, especially if your body is already under stress from caregiving.

If you use alcohol, do so responsibly. The key is moderation.

Have regular health checkups, especially for your blood pressure and cholesterol. Tap into the medical expertise of those who minister to your care receiver and ask questions about your own health concerns.

My Strategy: _____

_____

■ **CONTROL YOUR FEELINGS**

Your feelings are strongly influenced by the way you think and what you say to yourself. If you're an unhappy caregiver, it could be because you jump to conclusions, exaggerate your problems, and think in absolute terms like *"never"* and *"always."*

Listen to what you tell yourself. If a negative thought emerges from your subconscious, make a concerted effort to stop it. Then quickly substitute a positive message in its place. Change, *"I'll never be able to do it,"* to *"I'll do my very best."* If you stick to positive thoughts, you'll have more energy, increased productivity, a healthier self–image, and greater control over your caregiving responsibilities.

Control your feelings of guilt and shame. If you make a mistake, admit it. Then figure out how it happened and what you can do to keep from making the same mistake again. Don't let guilty thoughts fill your mind and sap your vitality. Move on with confidence and the knowledge that whatever you do next will not be affected by a past mistake.

Learn to recognize and understand your moods. They're conscious states of mind in which your emotions gain control of your behavior. Make them work for you, not against you. If you're in a lousy mood, change it before doing a caregiving task. If you can't change it, do something that won't affect your feelings toward your care receiver or your caregiving responsibilities.

Being angry is okay, but letting anger take over your behavior is not okay. Misdirected or bottled–up anger can be physically and emotionally detrimental to your well–being and can lead to caregiver abuse. Controlling your feelings may be one of the hardest things you've ever had to do, especially when you're exhausted or your care receiver has done something to get under your skin. Vent your anger in healthy ways, toward correctable situations and not at people.

Develop a personal support system in which you can vent the anger or frustration that pops up from time to time. Talk to your minister, priest, imam, or rabbi. Turn to a longtime friend. If there is no one else, then chop wood, go for a walk, or do as Thomas Jefferson suggested. *"When angry, count ten before you speak; if very angry, a hundred."*

My Strategy: _____

_____

■ MANAGE STRESS

The stress of caregiving does not in itself pose a serious threat to your health and happiness. It's your response to stress that causes burnout.

Control your stress by controlling your thoughts about caregiving. Think of yourself as having been selected–not shanghaied–into a role that carries with it a lot of personal responsibility and satisfaction. To think otherwise is folly. As the German philosopher Friedrich Nietzsche said, *"Nothing on earth consumes a man more quickly than the passion of resentment."*

Not all stress is negative, so you don't have to engage in stress–free activities to combat destructive stress. You can relieve the everyday stress of caregiving by pursuing substitute activities that create *positive* stress. Here are some examples you might consider if you have the time to do them.

- ✔ Sports: *golf, volleyball, racquetball, cross–country skiing.*
- ✔ Competitive bridge: *could be cutthroat!*
- ✔ The performing arts: *on stage before a critical audience.*
- ✔ Do–it–yourself remodeling: *ever try wallpapering?*

Control your stress through goal–setting and problem solving. Operate from a clear and consistent base. Be decisive and act quickly if it looks like things are starting to fall apart. Reach out for advice, look for lasting solutions, and form new action plans. If you assume that nothing will get done, nothing will.

Be realistic in your expectations. Plan a definite course of action, but accept change as a fact of life and be willing to live with it. Replace outmoded strategies when they no longer serve your needs or those of your care receiver.

Know what is expected of you, but don't try to accomplish unrealistic goals. Seek consensus with your care receiver and with family and friends over common goals and shared responsibilities. Try to resolve conflicts that can set one party against another.

Develop a sense of inner harmony by clarifying your beliefs and values. Find your source of spirituality through prayer, reading, meditation, contemplation, or attending formal religious services. Manage your stress as effectively as you manage your caregiving responsibilities.

My Strategy: _____

_____

■ COMMUNICATE

Speak up when things bother you. If you repress your concerns, you'll sap your energy, increase your frustration, and bring on negative stress.

Be realistic in your comments. Don't make light of your problems or exaggerate them beyond belief. Be diplomatic, and emphasize positive as well as negative points when you express your feelings.

Share your concerns with your care receiver. If the two of you work together, you can share your griefs and worries and develop common strategies for solving common problems. If your care receiver has trouble communicating, think up creative ways in which ideas can be expressed in writing, sign language, flash cards, or colored cubes.

Let people other than your care receiver know what you're going through. Negotiate a balance between social needs, work requirements, family responsibilities, and caregiving. If you can't get others to give care, at least let them help resolve your caregiving concerns.

Listen carefully to what others have to say to you. Confirm your interpretation of what you thought you heard by paraphrasing the message. Say, *"My understanding of what you're saying is..."*. If the interpretation is accurate, you've listened effectively to a well–stated point. If not, you've given the speaker another chance to clear up the confusion. Evaluate what has been said and then act accordingly.

The art of communicating is superbly expressed in this Cherokee Prayer: *"O Great Spirit help me always to speak the truth quietly, to listen with an open mind when others speak, and to remember the peace that may be found in silence."*

My Strategy: _____

_____

■ DEPERSONALIZE

Don't feel that everything that goes wrong with your care receiver or your caregiving situation is your fault. Keep an objective viewpoint and attribute to the disability or illness what is rightfully due. Don't carry an emotional burden that belongs someplace else.

You are not a failure if ...

... you continually strive to be a better caregiver.

... you seek training or professional help on how to cope with your emotions.

... you admit that caregiving is difficult or unpleasant and that you need respite from your responsibilities.

Accept who you are and set limits on what you can do. Establish realistic expectations, acceptable outcomes, and modest accomplishments. Do the best you can to make sure they're all realized. Keep in mind that you will not be able to handle every situation to perfection. Feel good about what you're able to do and know you did your best even when the results are less than satisfactory. Be careful not to second–guess yourself when things don't go the way they should. Immerse yourself in positive thoughts and avoid the risk of physical and mental exhaustion.

Be guided in your efforts by the words of the American author, Edward Everett Hale. *"I am only one, But still I am one. I cannot do everything, But still I can do something. And because I cannot do everything, I will do the something that I can do."*

My Strategy: _____

_____

■ SATISFY YOUR NEEDS

You must not allow yourself to be smothered by other people's demands or psychologically consumed by your caregiving responsibilities. Giving until it hurts is not a true measure of love. Protect your well–being by exercising, eating right, getting plenty of rest and having fun. Take time to understand and deal with feelings and needs that are uniquely yours.

Make a life of your own apart from caregiving, and do it without feeling guilty. Cultivate your strengths and eliminate your weaknesses. Join a support group. Try to find time to pursue a hobby or become a volunteer. Ask a social worker or health–care professional for suggestions. Do what you have to do to enhance your self–confidence and satisfy your needs.

Professionalize your caregiving role. Separate it from your home life, just as you would any other job. Set meaningful goals and strive for their completion. Step back from your caregiving at the end of the day, even if it's only for a short time. Give yourself some breathing room and strive to grow as an individual as well as a loving caregiver.

My Strategy: _____

_____

■   BUILD A SUPPORT SYSTEM

Supportive relationships provide much of what it takes to survive the rigors of caregiving. It's a proven fact that people who have support systems get along better than those who don't.

A support system provides a positive environment in which stress and frustration can be acknowledged, ventilated, clarified, and redirected. It can also take on a variety of forms and purposes. It can be a formalized group of people who share a common concern over a specific illness or disability, or it can be an informal network of family, friends, and co–workers who are willing to help where they can. In either case, a support system offers a comparison of strategies and a smorgasbord of help, humor, escape, rewards, comfort, and insight.

Track down appropriate support groups through newspapers, hospital social workers, community service agencies, or other health–care professionals. When you find a group that serves your needs, join it. Otherwise start one yourself. Attend the meetings and get involved in group activities. Draw on the knowledge and skill of your peers, and don't hesitate to offer your own suggestions.

Your introduction to a formal support group may be frightening, especially if you're meeting a group of people you've never seen before. They won't remain strangers for very long, because everyone will understand and appreciate what everybody else is going through. Just knowing that someone else is facing problems similar to yours will renew your energy and give you a whole new outlook on life.

Support goes both ways. As you gain confidence and support from people in your group, you in turn can reach out to others who need to know that they are not alone.

"Give what you have. To some it may be better than you dare to think." – Henry Wadsworth Longfellow.

My Strategy: _____

_____

■   **BUILD FRIENDSHIPS**

"Friendship improves happiness and abates misery by doubling our joy and dividing our grief." – Joseph Addison, English essayist.

One of the worst things that can happen when you become a caregiver is to lose contact with your friends. Friends provide a source of refuge and strength. You'll usually find them more than willing to listen, share your burden, and multiply your joy. Without friends, you can easily become isolated from social contact and subject to enormous stress.

Friendships take time and energy to develop and maintain. That's especially hard when so much of your attention is directed to your care receiver. You may feel too tired to spend time with friends, but it's absolutely essential to your well–being that you make the effort. You'll not only feel better, you'll erect another barrier against burnout.

Strive to maintain the warmth and comfort that comes from close, supportive relationships. Demonstrate a sincere interest in others and be willing to listen. Seek social relaxation as well as support from people who understand your situation and are willing to share with you on a regular basis.

Consider establishing or renewing ties with a church, synagogue, or other religious organization. You'll revive old friendships and establish new ones. Your rabbi, imam, priest, or minister will gladly provide support and comfort, and the organization may have a list of other resources that can help.

Take advantage of those rare occasions when you can find relief from caregiving, and do things with people you enjoy. Pursue a hobby that involves other people or attend discussion groups. You'll find it a lot easier to maintain your friendships when you are involved in activities that you have in common with your friends.

My Strategy: _____

_____

SUMMARY

You've gone through twenty–one strategies for preventing caregiver burnout. Hopefully, as you went through them, others came to mind and you wrote them down. If you added your ideas to the ones you found here, you should have a long list of things that will help maintain your positive approach toward caregiving. All you need now is a plan of action to put those ideas into practice. That's what you'll find in the final section.

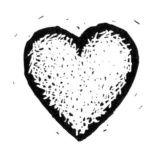

YOUR PLAN OF ACTION

Recall the definition of burnout that you read at the beginning. It's a state of physical, emotional, and psychological exhaustion that is accompanied by a shift in attitude from positive and caring to negative and uncaring.

You have seen what causes burnout, and you have several strategies for coping with it. Now is the time to put it all together and create a plan of action. Here are eight specific steps you can take right now to prevent caregiver burnout or restore your commitment to caregiving if you've gotten a little close to the fire.

1. RECOGNIZE YOUR BURNOUT POTENTIAL

Ask yourself the following two key questions to see if you're a candidate for burnout.

►   *"How many times have I found myself on the verge of giving up, only to pull back with a renewed attitude toward caregiving?"*

►   *"How many times have I avoided certain caregiving duties because I knew they'd make me tired, angry or frustrated?"*

If you can recall instances where your attitude shifted because of caregiving stress, then you must recognize that you are a potential candidate for burnout. If you don't recognize that now, then you're likely to run into problems later on.

2.   GET THE FACTS

Take inventory of your behavior. How has your attitude toward caregiving affected your health, energy, finances, and self–image? How has it affected others, including family, friends, and your care receiver? What specific incidents have triggered negative attitudes? What emotions, like fear, anger, guilt, or impatience, have fueled your frustration?

Figure out where the soft spots are, then review the preventative strategies in this book and take positive steps to protect yourself from burnout.

3.   KNOW YOUR JOB

Meet with your care receiver, family and friends to confirm your caregiving responsibilities. Verify your role with social workers and other professionals, as well as members of your support group.

Know what your physical and mental strengths and weaknesses are and don't be afraid to set limits on what you can do. If others suggest that you could do more, explain to them that going beyond those limits could lead to burnout. Make sure you and everyone else knows what the consequences would be if they lost you as an effective caregiver.

4. HAVE HOPE

"In all things it is better to hope than despair." This advice, by the German philosopher Johann Goethe, applies to every caregiver.

Know what you can realistically expect as a caregiver. Cast aside pie–in–the–sky aspirations that can never be reached, but don't give up hope. Hope can keep you from being held hostage by your care receiver's illness or disability. Hope provides the encouragement you need to thrive in a frustrating environment.

Give the best you can and the best will come back to you.

5. DEVELOP NEW TOOLS FOR COPING

Recognize the need for better strategies and seek them out wherever you can. Read books, listen to self–help tapes, and borrow ideas from others. Develop an arsenal of effective coping techniques that will get you through the darkest hours. Improve the range and quality of strategies that have served you well in the past, like good listening and clear communication. Don't get stuck in the worst of what is, but work toward the best of what can be.

6. ASK FOR HELP

Pay close attention to the early symptoms of burnout. Stop them if you can, but if they are more than you can handle, then waste no time in seeking outside help. You can find help from spiritual sources or from friends, family members, organizations, agencies or formal support groups. You can also get help from your rabbi, imam, priest, or pastor or from counselors, psychologists or psycho-therapists. Figure out what you need, then be aggressive in seeking it.

There are many other caregivers just like you doing the same kinds of things for people they love or care about. The knowledge and experience they have gained over the years can provide tremendous support for those who need it. It's a network you can easily tie into.

7. LIVE ONE DAY AT A TIME

Have reasonable and consistent expectations, but don't try to take gigantic leaps unless you're a trapeze artist. Consider author Leo Hauser's maxim, *"By the yard it's hard, by the inch it's a cinch."*

8. DO IT NOW!

Plan gradual improvements instead of sudden overnight changes. Focus your energy on today's challenges and stop worrying about problems that may never develop.

You've taken the first step toward preventing caregiver burnout by reading this book. By now, you should know about the effects of burnout, what causes it, and how to prevent it from taking over your life. You've seen how it affects other people's lives, and you've entertained a number of questions that have probed your thoughts about its effect on you. Now it's time to recover your spark and develop some positive intentions.

Others are waiting for you. It's time to act. Do it!

AVAILABLE RESOURCES

It would be impossible to provide an up–to–date list of available resources for every area of the country. Or for that matter, other countries besides the United States where caregivers are found. What is provided here is a generic list of people, agencies, and organizations that can provide help when the need arises.

Use this list as an entry to your phone book, community service agency, or support group, and build a list of your own. Just be sure to share it with the next caregiver you meet. There is no one who needs help more than one who has no where to turn.

Hospitals
Senior centers
Support groups
Legal aid services
State units on aging
Volunteer programs
Ombudsman services
In–house respite care
Home chore services
Home health services
Home delivered meals
Housekeeping services
Area agencies on aging
Veteran's affairs offices
Senior citizen's services
Adult daycare programs
Out–of–home respite care

County extension services
Caregiver Resource Centers
Community health services
County public health nurses
Economic assistance agencies
Social Security district offices
State human services agencies
County human service agencies
Illness and disability associations
Information and referral agencies
Mental health and counseling agencies
Illness and disability treatment centers
Social service agencies sponsored by governmental bodies
Social service agencies affiliated with church or association

There are many agencies that provide support in specialized areas dealing with diseases like Alzheimer's, Parkinson's, or diabetes. Many others offer help to people who have ailments related to parts of the body such as heart, lungs, or kidneys.

You might start by calling the United Way, the National Council on Aging, the American Association of Retired Persons, or the Eldercare Information and Referral Service at 1-800-677-1116.

The thing to remember is that *you are not alone.* There are millions of people all over the world who understand your problems and are willing to help.

INDEX

INDEX

ABOUT THE AUTHOR

James R. Sherman is the author and publisher of 17 books, including the national bestseller, *Stop Procrastinating—DO IT!*, which has sold over 350,000 copies. His books have been reproduced on cassette tape, marketed worldwide, and translated into Chinese, French, German, Hungarian, Japanese, and Spanish. Dr. Sherman has appeared on the NBC TODAY show as well as on regional and local radio and television programs. His self–help articles have appeared in national, regional, and local publications. His lively and entertaining talks about success and procrastination have rounded out his publishing career.

Born and raised in southwestern Minnesota, Dr. Sherman received his bachelor's and master's degrees from the University of Colorado and his doctorate from the University of Northern Colorado. Following positions as Assistant Professor of Educational Psychology at the University of Minnesota and Assistant Chancellor of the Minnesota Community College System, Jim spent seven years as a management consultant to colleges and universities across the country. He established Pathway Books in 1979 and has devoted full time to his writing, speaking, and publishing efforts ever since. He does much of his writing at his cabin adjacent to the Boundary Waters Canoe Area Wilderness in northern Minnesota.

He now brings his extensive caregiving experience to his writing in a new 12–book, self–help series for caregivers.

ABOUT THE SENIOR EDITOR

Merlene Sherman completed graduate studies in nursing home and hospital administration at the University of Minnesota and has worked in geriatrics for 20 years. She worked extensively with caregivers while developing and directing two adult daycare programs in Minneapolis. She is internationally known for her programs in workplace wellness and is the author of two health promotion books, *Wellness in the Workplace* and *Health Strategies for Working Women.*

Merlene and Jim have been married for 37 years. For over 13 years they were caregivers to both sets of parents, now deceased. They have three adult sons and now enjoy playing with, doting upon, and overfeeding their grandchildren.

THE CAREGIVER SURVIVAL SERIES

Preventing Caregiver Burnout

Caregivers who work long, hard hours under constant emotional pressure can very easily lose their motivation and commitment to caregiving. This dynamic book responds to that threat by describing what burnout is, what causes it, and what effect it can have on a caregiver's vitality. Best of all, it presents an extensive list of easy–to–follow procedures for preventing burnout and maintaining an optimistic outlook toward caregiving.

Creative Caregiving

This book inspires caregivers to develop creative ways of relieving the most maddening aspects of caregiving. It provides a wealth of innovative techniques that show caregivers how to work smarter, not harder, and make the most of precious free time. Once they read this book, caregivers will wonder how they ever got along without it.

Positive Caregiver Attitudes

A "must" book for any caregiver whose back is against the wall. It's loaded with down–to–earth strategies for developing and maintaining positive attitudes toward care receivers, caregiving, and life in general. The book identifies the source of negative feelings and illustrates the destructive effect negative attitudes can produce if left unresolved. It provides a vital safeguard for any caregiving relationship.

The Magic of Humor in Caregiving

This resourceful book can provide tremendous benefits and tickle a caregiver's funny bone at the same time. The well–established healing benefits of laughter in reducing stress and tension are clearly explained. The book also shows how playfulness can be used to increase personal effectiveness and promote wellness. It leaves no doubt that laughter is often the best medicine a caregiver can use.

The Caregiver's Guide to Problem Solving

This eye–opening book helps caregivers identify problems, determine their root causes, explore alternative strategies, make realistic choices, and implement effective solutions to caregiving problems. It's an indispensable tool that takes the guesswork out of day–to–day decision making and makes the hard job of caregiving much easier. No caregiver should without it.

Conquering Caregiver Fears

This dynamite book pinpoints the sources of fear, anxiety, guilt, and depression, and tells why they exist. It outfits caregivers with surefire methods for controlling anxiety, building courage, and maintaining the self–confidence they need to conquer the destructive forces that often accompany and threaten caregiving. This is a no–nonsense manual that will stand up under years of repeated use.

Strengthening the Caregiver Family

Holding a family together and dealing with interpersonal conflicts is a challenge for many caregivers. This timely book outlines the sources of family conflict, then puts forth an ample supply of time–tested solutions for building and maintaining family harmony. It empowers caregivers to tackle unmet needs, sibling rivalries, generational differences, caregiving role disputes and other difficulties with confidence and conviction.

Love, Companionship and Caregiving

This revealing book helps caregivers recognize the physical and emotional challenges that interfere with normal expressions of love, affection, and companionship. Its down–to–earth strategies help caregivers deal with the physical and emotional burdens that frequently accompany caregiving. Readers gain a clear perspective on how to recognize problems, overcome obstacles, and meet basic personal needs while in a caregiving relationship. Creative suggestions tell how to maintain tender, intimate relationships and turn difficult moments into priceless memories.

Health Strategies for Active Caregivers

A made–to–order book that highlights the special health and fitness needs of caregivers and shows how those needs can be satisfied within the caregiving environment. It provides detailed instructions for staying in excellent condition while meeting the unrelenting demands of the caregiver role. Wellness strategies for nutrition, exercise, sleep, and stress reduction show caregivers how to maintain a healthy lifestyle.

The Caregiver's Need for People

This candid book focuses on the caregiver's need for extensive human interaction, not just with the care receiver, but with family, friends, health care professionals, and other caregivers. It stresses the importance of making new friends and keeping existing friendships intact. The book provides an ample supply of techniques for enhancing social contacts and opportunities. This book is standard equipment for anyone who is involved in an activity that is as people–intensive as caregiving.

The Caregiver's Planning Guide

Caregivers, in almost every case, soon discover that they must respond quickly and effectively to the never–ending demands of an unpredictable future. This superb planning guide helps clarify the caregivers present position, helps them determine where they want to be in the future, and shows them what they have to do to get there. It provides an abundance of time–proven procedures for developing workable plans for taking the drudgery out of caregiving.

Financial Fitness for Caregivers

This user–friendly book provides an in–depth look at the financial demands that often overwhelm unsuspecting caregivers. It's loaded with cost–effective suggestions for alleviating financial stress, discovering new sources of funds and meeting special caregiving needs. Every caregiver who has had to face the continuous rise in health–care costs will find this book to be an effective weapon against financial worries.

HOW TO ORDER

Now you can build a library of outstanding self-help books for caregivers with no hassle and at an unbelievably low price.

The subject matter of the 12 books in the *Caregiver Survival Series* covers some of the major concerns of millions of people just like you. Each book gives you an easy-to-understand explanation of why you're having problems. They also give you clear, concise guidelines for eliminating those problems and turning your life as a caregiver into a compelling and rewarding experience.

The books are easy to come by. Just call us at 612-377-1521 or make a copy of the order form on the next page and send it to our Golden Valley address. Tell us how many copies you want of each title, add 6.5% for Minnesota sales tax and an appropriate amount for shipping, and include your check or money order. We'll have your books in the mail within 24-48 hours. If you order more than 10 books, we'll bill you for the actual shipping costs.

The books in the *Caregiver Survival Series* are guaranteed to make you a better caregiver. If-for any reason-you're not satisfied, send your books back, and you'll get an immediate refund. We'll still keep your name on our mailing list so you won't miss out on any news about future books in the series.

ORDER FORM

Title	Price	No.	Cost
Preventing Caregiver Burnout	$ 7.95	x _____	= $ _____
Creative Caregiving	$ 7.95	x _____	= $ _____
Positive Caregiver Attitudes	$ 7.95	x _____	= $ _____
The Magic of Humor in Caregiving	$ 7.95	x _____	= $ _____
The Caregiver's Guide to Problem Solving	$ 7.95	x _____	= $ _____
Conquering Caregiver Fears	$ 7.95	x _____	= $ _____
Strengthening the Caregiver Family	$ 7.95	x _____	= $ _____
Love, Compassion, and Caregiving	$ 7.95	x _____	= $ _____
Health Strategies for Active Caregivers	$ 7.95	x _____	= $ _____
The Caregiver's Need for People	$ 7.95	x _____	= $ _____
The Caregiver's Planning Guide	$ 7.95	x _____	= $ _____
Financial Fitness for Caregivers	$ 7.95	x _____	= $ _____

Shipping Charges

Subtotal $ _____

1 copy   = $1.50
2–5 copies = $ 2.00
6-10 copies = $ 2.50
10+ copies = actual

Adjustment $ _____

Shipping charges $ _____

NET DUE (30 days) $ _____

* These three books are currently available. The remaining books in the series will be completed in 1995 and 1996.

SHIP TO (Please type or print clearly)

NAME: _____

ADDRESS–1: _____

ADDRESS-2: _____

CITY/STATE/ZIP: _____

PHONE: _____ DATE: _____

═══

BILL TO (If different from above)

NAME: _____

ADDRESS–1: _____

ADDRESS–2: _____

CITY/STATE/ZIP: _____

PHONE: _____ DATE: _____

Pathway Books
700 Parkview Terrace
Golden Valley, MN 55416
(612) 377–1521